# KIDNEY STONES

Kidney Stones: Guide On Kidney Stone, Symptoms, Causes, Natural Remedies Treatment, Prevention

**Mary F. Phipps**

**Table of Contents**

CHAPTER ONE ........................... 2

KIDNEY STONES ....................... 2

Different kinds of kidney stones .. 3

   Calcium ................................. 3

   Uric destructive ..................... 4

   Struvite ................................. 5

   Cystine .................................. 5

Incidental effects and signs of a kidney stone ............................. 6

Different results of kidney stones can include: .................... 7

Purposes behind kidney stones 8

Other bet factors include: ......... 9

CHAPTER TWO ......................... 11

HOW KIDNEY STONES ARE MANAGED ................................ 11

Other treatment decisions: ......... 11

    Drugs ........................................ 11

    Lithotripsy .............................. 13

    Ureteroscopy ......................... 14

    Torture the chiefs ................... 15

    Testing for and diagnosing kidney stones ......................... 16

CHAPTER THREE......................19

PASSING A KIDNEY STONE.....19

    Stages.......................................19

    Stage 1:....................................19

    Stage 2:....................................20

    Stage 3:....................................20

    Stage 4: ...................................21

    Time it expect to elapse a kidney stone .........................................21

    Guidelines to prevent kidney stones ......................................22

Food sources that can cause kidney stones ..........................24

Foods assortments that to restrict or avoid:......................24

When to see a subject matter expert ........................................26

Kidney Stone eating routine:..28

CHAPTER FOUR........................30

WHAT TO EAT AND DRINK.....30

Stay hydrated ..........................30

Up your citrus utilization .......30

Eat heaps of calcium (and vitamin D) ............................... 31

Food and drinks to avoid on a kidney stone eating schedule ..... 33

Limit salt ................................. 33

Cut down your animal protein affirmation ............................ 34

Know about oxalates ............... 35

Food assortments high in oxalate include: ....................... 36

Avoid drinking colas ............... 36

Tips for a kidney stone eating routine..................................38

Tips that will help include: .....39

Home Answers for Kidney Stones: ..................................40

CHAPTER FIVE .........................41

HOW WE VET BRANDS AND THINGS......................................41

Staying hydrated is fundamental ................................................41

1. Water ...................................43

2. Lemon juice.........................44

3. Basil juice ...........................45

4. Squeezed apple vinegar.......47

5. Celery juice..........................49

## CHAPTER SIX ...........................52

## ALTERNATE WAY VET BRANDS AND THINGS ..........................52

1. Pomegranate juice ...............52

2. Kidney bean stock ...............54

Other standard fixes................55

3. Dandelion ...........................55

4. Wheatgrass juice .................58

5. Horsetail ............................60

When to see a subject matter expert ........................................61

The primary concern ..............62

CHAPTER SEVEN ......................66

STRATEGIES FOR PREVENTING KIDNEY STONES ......................66

Kidney stone expectation .......66

The best strategy to hinder kidney stones typically ............67

1. Stay hydrated ......................68

2. Eat more calcium-rich food sources ....................................69

3. Eat less sodium ................... 70

Food assortments renowned for being high in sodium include: .71

4. Eat less oxalate-rich food sources ..................................... 73

Food sources high in oxalates are: ......................................... 73

5. Eat less animal protein ....... 74

You should endeavor to confine or avoid: ................................. 75

6. Avoid L-ascorbic corrosive upgrades ................................. 75

7. Explore local fixes ................76

CHAPTER EIGHT........................77

WAYS OF THWARTING KIDNEY STONES WITH MEDICATION ..77

1. Till your doctor about the medications you're at this point ..................................................77

A part of these medications are: ..................................................78

2. Letting your doctor about security medicines ...................79

For example: ...........................80

Will kidney stones cause gastrointestinal incidental effects? ...................................82

Torture ...................................83

Nausea...................................83

Heaving ..................................84

Expected gastrointestinal intricacies of kidney stones ....84

Prickly entrail condition .........85

Entrail obstacle .......................86

Might gastrointestinal issues anytime cause kidney stones? 86

Detachment of the entrails .....87

CHAPTER NINE .......................88

PROVOCATIVE INSIDE CONTAMINATION.....................88

Stomach operations................88

Other kidney stones incidental effects .......................................89

When to contact an expert if you expect you have kidney stones ...................................................90

Frequently looked for explanation on certain things .92

Can kidney stones impact strong releases...................................93

What GI issues can cause kidney stones?......................................93

What GI issues can kidney stones cause? ..........................94

Could kidney stones cause IBS? ................................................94

# CHAPTER ONE

## KIDNEY STONES

Kidney stones, or renal calculi, are solid masses made of diamonds. Kidney stones by and large start in your kidneys. In any case, they can encourage wherever along your urinary bundle, which contains **these parts:**

- kidneys
- ureters
- bladder
- urethra

Kidney stones can be a troublesome clinical issue. The explanations behind kidney stones vacillate according to the sort of stones.

## Different kinds of kidney stones

### Calcium

Calcium stones are the most widely recognized. They're regularly made of calcium oxalate, but they can include calcium phosphate or maleate.

Eating less oxalate-rich food assortments can diminish your bet of encouraging this kind of stone. **High-oxalate food assortments include:**

- potato chips

- peanuts
- chocolate
- spinach

Regardless, in spite of the way that some kidney stones are made of calcium, getting adequate calcium in your eating routine can hold stones back from molding.

**Uric destructive**

This kind of kidney stone is the second commonly typical. They can occur in people with gout, diabetes, bulkiness, and various types of metabolic issue.

This sort of stone makes when pee is unreasonably acidic. An eating routine rich in pureness can build pee's acidic level. Purina is a boring substance in animal proteins, similar to fish, shellfish, and meats.

## Struvite

This kind of stone is found generally in people with urinary bundle defilements (UTIs). These stones can be colossal and cause urinary deterrent.

Struvite stones result from a kidney tainting. Treating a secret sickness can prevent the improvement of struvite stones.

## Cystine

Around 1 out of 7,000 people generally speaking get cystine

kidney stones. They occur in a wide range of individuals who have the genetic issue cystinuria.

With this kind of stone, cystine a destructive that happens typically in the body spills from the kidneys into the pee.

## Incidental effects and signs of a kidney stone

Kidney stones can cause outrageous torture. Symptoms of kidney stones may not occur until the stone begins to drop down the ureters. This outrageous disturbance is called renal colic. You might have torture on one side of your back or mid-locale.

In men, anguish could send to the groin district. The exacerbation of renal colic goes this way and that anyway can be phenomenal. People with renal colic will as a rule is worrisome.

**Different results of kidney stones can include:**

- blood in the pee (red, pink, or hearty shaded pee)
- spewing
- squeamishness
- stained or foul pee
- chills
- fever
- progressive need to pee

- peeing humble amounts of pee

By virtue of a little kidney stone, you probably won't have any exacerbation or secondary effects as the stone goes through your urinary plot.

## Purposes behind kidney stones

Kidney stones are most likely going to occur in people between the ages of 20 and 50.

Different components can fabricate your bet of cultivating a stone. In the US, white people will undoubtedly have kidney stones than People of variety.

Sex similarly expects a section. A greater number of men than women cultivate kidney stones, according to the Public Underpinning of Diabetes and Stomach related and Kidney Sicknesses (NIDDK).

A past loaded up with kidney stones can fabricate your bet. So does a family foundation of kidney stones.

**Other bet factors include:**
- absence of hydration
- weight
- an eating routine with raised levels of protein, salt, or glucose

- hyperparathyroidism condition
- gastric diversion an operation
- searing stomach infections that increase calcium digestion
- Taking drugs, for instance, triamterene diuretics, anti seizure meds, and calcium-based corrosive neutralizers.

# CHAPTER TWO

## HOW KIDNEY STONES ARE MANAGED

Treatment is specially designed by the kind of stone. Pee can be focused on and stones assembled for evaluation.

Drinking six to eight glasses of water a day increases pee stream. People who are dried out or have outrageous ailment and heaving might require intravenous fluids.

**Other treatment decisions:**

### Drugs

Assist with uneasiness might require narcotic medications. The presence of sickness requires therapy with hostile to microbial. **Various drugs include:**

- allopurinol (Zyloprim) for uric destructive stones
- thiamine diuretics to thwart calcium stones from forming
- sodium bicarbonate or sodium citrate to make the pee less acidi
- phosphorus deals with prevent calcium stones from outlining
- ibuprofen (Advil) for torture
- acetaminophen (Tylenol) for torture

- naproxen sodium (Aleve) for torture

**Lithotripsy**

Extracorporeal shock wave lithotripsy uses sound waves to isolate tremendous stones so they might even more at any point successfully pass down the ureters into your bladder.

This method can be abnormal and may require light sedation. It can cause expanding on the mid-locale and back and depleting around the kidney and nearby organs.

Tunnel an operation (percutaneous nephrolithotomy)

An expert eliminates the stones through a little passage point in your back. An individual could require this **procedure when:**

- the stone causes obstruction and infection or is hurting the kidneys
- the stone has become excessively immense to try and contemplate passing
- torture can't be made due

**Ureteroscopy**

Right when a stone is caught in the ureter or bladder, your PCP could use an instrument called a ureteroscope to kill it.

A little wire with a camera joined is inserted into the urethra and passed into the bladder. The expert then, uses a little nook to get the stone and dispense with it. The stone is then transported off the exploration place for assessment.

### Torture the chiefs

Passing a kidney stone can cause torture and pain. Your PCP could propose taking an over-the-counter pain reliever, similar to acetaminophen or ibuprofen, to help with reducing secondary effects.

For serious distress, your essential consideration doctor may moreover recommend a narcotic or imbue a quieting drug, similar to ketorolac (Toradol).

Other typical fixes may in like manner give transient assistance from secondary effects, including scouring or shower or applying a warming pad to the influenced district.

## Testing for and diagnosing kidney stones

Finish of kidney stones requires an all out prosperity history assessment and a genuine test. **Various tests include:**

- blood tests for calcium, phosphorus, uric destructive, and electrolytes
- blood urea nitrogen (BUN) and creatinine to assess kidney working
- urinalysis to check for valuable stones, microorganisms, blood, and white cells
- evaluation of passed stones to choose their sort

The going with tests can block **obstruction:**

- stomach X-radiates
- intravenous pyelogram (IVP)
- retrograde pyelogram

- ultrasound of the kidney (the leaned toward test)
- X-beam clear of the mid-district and kidneys
- stomach CT look at

The distinction variety used in the CT check and the IVP can impact kidney ability. Regardless, in people with common kidney capacity, this isn't a concern.

There are a couple of medications that can extend the potential for kidney hurt connected with the variety. Guarantee your radiologist acknowledges about any medications you're taking.

# CHAPTER THREE

## PASSING A KIDNEY STONE

Passing a kidney stone is a cycle that consistently occurs in stages throughout a period of a portion of a month.

### Stages

Here are the stages that happen while passing a kidney stone.

**Stage 1:** After a kidney stone has molded, you could experience fits as your kidneys endeavor to push out the stone. This can cause outrageous anguish in your back or side, which could go this way and that in waves.

**Stage 2:** During this stage, the stone enters the ureter, which is the chamber that relates the kidneys to the bladder. Dependent upon the size of the stone, this stage can in like manner create uproars of distress and outrageous strain.

**Stage 3:** At the point when the stone has shown up at the bladder, a huge piece of the disturbance will subside. In any case, you could feel an extended strain in the bladder and a need to pee even more a significant part of the time. On occasion, the stone may momentarily slow down at the send off of the urethra, which could block the movement of pee.

**Stage 4:** The last stage happens once the stone has shown up at the urethra. During this stage, you need to push hard to pass the kidney stone with the pee through the send off of the urethra.

## Time it expect to elapse a kidney stone

What amount of time that it requires to pass a kidney stone can change dependent upon the size of the stone. Generally, little stones can go through the peek inside 1 fourteen days, every now and again with close to no treatment.

Of course, greater stones could require 2-3 weeks to go through the kidneys and into the bladder.

Stones that don't pass on their own in something like a month normally require clinical treatment.

## Guidelines to prevent kidney stones

Real hydration is a crucial preventive measure. It's recommended to drink adequate fluid to pass somewhere near 2.5 liters Wellspring of pee consistently. Extending how much pee you pass helps flush the kidneys.

You can substitute pop, lemon-lime pop and natural item squeeze for water to help you with growing your fluid confirmation. Accepting the stones are associated with low citrate levels, citrate juices could help with preventing the advancement of stones.

Eating oxalate-rich food sources with a few restrictions and diminishing your confirmation of salt and animal proteins can moreover cut down your bet of kidney stones.

Your essential consideration doctor could prescribe medications to help with thwarting the improvement of calcium and uric destructive stones. If you've had a kidney stone or you're in peril for a kidney stone, talk with your PCP and look at the best procedures for countering.

### Food sources that can cause kidney stones

As well as drinking more water, making acclimations to your eating routine could in like manner help with thwarting kidney stones.

### Foods assortments that to restrict or avoid:

- meat

- chicken
- pork
- organ meats
- fish
- shellfish
- eggs
- milk
- cheddar
- yogurt
- taken care of meats
- modest food
- frozen feasts
- impactful goodies

Animal proteins like meat, poultry, fish, and dairy things can fabricate levels of uric destructive in your pee and addition the bet of making kidney stones.

## When to see a subject matter expert

A significant part of the time, little kidney stones can pass isolated and require no treatment.

Accepting for the time being that you're prepared to manage your disturbance with non-doctor prescribed prescriptions and have no signs of tainting or outrageous secondary effects like nausea or disgorging, you may not need treatment.

Regardless, accepting you experience any of the going with

aftereffects, you should search without a doubt fire clinical **thought:**

- blood in the pee
- fever
- chills
- obscure or rotten pee
- regurgitating
- serious torture in your back or side
- torture or consuming when you pee
- inconvenience peeing

In case you can't see your essential consideration doctor, you should go to the ER to seek treatment.

Expecting that you have redundant kidney stones, you should talk with your essential consideration doctor, whether or not your incidental effects resolve without treatment.

Your PCP can help with encouraging an arrangement to thwart kidney stones from molding and protect against long stretch snares.

**Kidney Stone eating routine:**
Kidney stones in the urinary bundle are formed in more than one manner. Calcium can get together with engineered materials, similar to oxalate or

phosphorous, in the pee. This can happen expecting these substances become so engaged that they solidify. Kidney stones can similarly be achieved by an improvement of uric destructive. Uric destructive advancement is achieved by the processing of protein. Your urinary plot wasn't planned to areas of strength for eliminate, so it's nothing surprising that kidney stones are extraordinarily challenging to pass. Luckily, they can commonly be avoided through diet.

## CHAPTER FOUR

### WHAT TO EAT AND DRINK

In case you're endeavoring to avoid kidney stones, what you eat and drink is essentially pretty much as critical as what you shouldn't eat and drink. Here are huge overall rules to recollect.

### Stay hydrated

Fluids, especially water, help to debilitate the manufactured substances that design stones. Endeavor to drink something like 12 glasses of water a day.

### Up your citrus utilization

Citrus regular item, and their juice, can help lessen or block the game plan of stones as a result of typically happening citrate. Incredible wellsprings of citrus consolidate lemons, oranges, and grapefruit.

## Eat heaps of calcium (and vitamin D)

Expecting your calcium confirmation is low, oxalate levels could rise. It's alluring over get your calcium from food, rather than from supplements, as these have been associated with kidney stone turn of events. Incredible wellsprings of calcium integrate milk, yogurt, curds, and various kinds of cheeses. Veggie lover wellsprings of calcium integrate vegetables, calcium-set tofu, dull green vegetables, nuts, seeds, and blackstrap molasses. If you could manage without the kind of cow's milk, then again, if it can't help contradicting you, endeavor sans lactose milk, supported soy milk, or goat's milk. In like manner try to recollect food sources high for vitamin D consistently. Vitamin D helps the body with holding more calcium. Various food sources are fortified with this supplement. It's moreover found in oily fishes, similar to salmon, mushrooms, and cheddar.

## Food and drinks to avoid on a kidney stone eating schedule

### Limit salt

High sodium levels in the body can propel calcium improvement in pee. Do whatever it takes not to add salt to food, and really take a gander at the names on dealt with food sources to see how much sodium they contain. Modest food can be high in sodium, yet so can standard bistro food. Right when you're able, ask that no salt be added to anything that you demand on a menu. Furthermore, see what you drink. A couple of vegetable juices are high in sodium.

## Cut down your animal protein affirmation

Numerous wellsprings of protein, similar to red meat, pork, chicken, poultry, and eggs, increase how much uric destructive you produce. Eating a ton of protein moreover diminishes a compound in pee called citrate. Citrate's liability is to hinder the improvement of kidney stones. Choices rather than animal protein integrate quinoa, tofu (bean curd), hummus, chia seeds, and Greek yogurt. Since protein is critical for the most part prosperity, inspect the sum you should eat everyday with your PCP.

**Know about oxalates**

Eat oxalates cautiously. Food assortments high in this substance could grow plan of kidney stones. If you've recently had kidney stones, you could wish to diminish or take out oxalates from your eating routine completely. If you're endeavoring to avoid kidney stones, check with your essential consideration doctor to conclude whether limiting these food varieties is adequate. In case you really eat food assortments containing oxalates, reliably try to eat or drink a calcium source with them. This will help the oxalate with confining to the calcium during digestion, before it can show up at your kidneys.

### Food assortments high in oxalate include:

- chocolate
- beets
- nuts
- tea
- rhubarb
- spinach
- Swiss chard
- sweet potatoes

### Avoid drinking colas

Cola is high in phosphate, another compound which can propel the course of action of kidney stones. Lessening or crash added sugar utilization added sugars can't avoid being sugars and syrups that are added to deal with food sources and drinks. Added sucrose and added fructose could assemble your bet of kidney stones. Look out for how much sugar you eat, in took care of food sources, similar to cake, in natural item, in soft drink pops, and in juices. Other typical added sugar names integrate corn syrup, cemented fructose, honey, agave nectar, hearty hued rice syrup, and unadulterated sugar.

## Tips for a kidney stone eating routine

Having kidney stones fabricates your bet of getting them again with the exception of assuming you really work to hinder them. This suggests ingesting medications prescribed to you hence, and watching what you eat and drink.

Expecting you right currently have stones, your PCP will run characteristic tests, to sort out what type you have. They will then, embrace a specific eating routine arrangement for you, for instance, the Scramble Diet.

**Tips that will help include:**

- drink something like twelve glasses of water everyday
- eat citrus natural items, similar to orange
- eat a calcium-rich food at each blowout, something like multiple times every day
- limit your affirmation of animal protein
- eat less salt, added sugar, and things containing high fructose corn syrup
- avoid food assortments and relishes high oxalates and phosphates

- Avoid eating or drinking anything which dries out you, similar to alcohol.

## Home Answers for Kidney Stones:

We integrate things we accept are useful for our perusers. If you buy through joins on this page, we could get a little commission Here's our collaboration.

# CHAPTER FIVE

## HOW WE VET BRANDS AND THINGS

Staying hydrated can help with passing kidney stones faster. Certain substances, including squeezed apple vinegar and lemon juice, may help with dissolving kidney stones, making them clearer to pass.

### Staying hydrated is fundamental

Drinking a great deal of fluids is a crucial piece of passing kidney stones and holding new stones back from outlining. Not at all does the liquid flush out harms; anyway it similarly helps move stones and coarseness through your urinary part.

Notwithstanding the way that water alone may be adequate to take care of business, adding explicit trimmings might be productive.

Talk with an expert before getting everything going with any of the home fixes recorded underneath. They can study whether these techniques are fitting for you then again if they could incite additional bothersome effects.

Make sure to drink one 8-ounce glass of water following drinking any carefully prepared fix. This can help with moving the trimmings through your structure.

If you're pregnant or breastfeeding, do whatever it takes not to use any fixes. An expert can choose if a juice could cause coincidental impacts for you or your kid.

### 1. Water

While passing a stone, expanding your water confirmation can help with speeding up the collaboration. Gain ground toward 12 glasses of water every day as opposed to the norm.

At the point when the stone passes, you should continue to

drink 8 to 12 glasses of water consistently. Drying out is one of the major bet factors for kidney stones, and the last thing you want is for more to outline. Center around the shade of your pee. It should be an incredibly light, light yellow. Dull yellow pee means that parchedness.

**2. Lemon juice**

You can add recently squeezed lemons to your water as often as you like. Lemons contain citrate, which is an engineered that hinders calcium stones from molding. Citrate can in like manner separate little stones, allowing them to pass even more easily.

A great deal of lemon juice would probably be supposed to have a tremendous effect, but some could help a little.

Lemon juice enjoys different other health advantages. For example, it upsets microorganism's turn of events and gives L-ascorbic corrosive.

### 3. Basil juice

Basil is overflowing with supplements. This fix has been involved generally Focal point for stomach related and combustible issues.

There are cell fortifications and quieting experts in basil juice, so it could stay aware of kidney prosperity. Nevertheless, there's little verification to help this fix.

To endeavor it, use new or dried basil gives to make a tea and drink a couple of cups every day. You may similarly crush new basil in a juicer or add it to a smoothie.

It's not known whether basil juice is safeguarded to drink in colossal sums, or over longer time spans. Without more investigation, the long effects stay unclear.

Notwithstanding the way that there's small investigation on how fruitful basil is for kidney stones, it has against oxidative and quieting properties.

**4. Squeezed apple vinegar**
Squeezed apple vinegar contains acidic destructive. Acidic destructive helpers separate kidney stones.

As well as flushing out the kidneys, squeezed apple vinegar could help with working with torture achieved by the stones.

One lab examination found that squeezed apple vinegar was convincing in reducing the game plan of kidney stones. Nevertheless, more examinations are supposed to see whether vinegar altogether influences kidney stones inside the human body.

To endeavor this fix, add 2 tablespoons of squeezed apple vinegar to 6 to 8 ounces of drinking water.

You shouldn't consume more than one 8-ounce glass of this mix every day. You can in like manner sprinkle squeezed apple vinegar onto servings of leafy greens or add it to your main serving of leafy greens dressing.

If ingested in greater aggregates, squeezed apple vinegar can cause issues, for instance, damage to tooth polish, acid reflux, and sore throat.

People with diabetes should rehearse alert while drinking this mix. Screen your glucose levels circumspectly throughout the span of the day.

You shouldn't drink this mix if you're taking certain prescriptions, including insulin or diuretics like spironolactone (Aldactone).

### 5. Celery juice

Celery is used in customary medications as an answer for help with kidney stones.

One examination found that female individuals with kidney stones ate less celery on ordinary than female individuals without kidney stones.

Likewise, a recent report in rodents found that celery separate helped separate kidney stones. Blend somewhere around one celery stems with water, and drink the juice.

Like other plant removes, it's useful for celery to associate with various solutions or meds, which could cause bothersome effects. It's for each situation best to check with an expert preceding endeavoring new fixes.

# CHAPTER SIX

## ALTERNATE WAY VET BRANDS AND THINGS

### 1. Pomegranate juice

Pomegranate juice has been used from now onward, indefinitely a truly significant time-frame to additionally foster in everyday kidney capacity. It will flush stones and various toxins from your system. It's stacked with cell fortifications, which help with keeping the kidneys sound and may have an impact in preventing kidney stones from making.

It moreover cuts down your pee's destructiveness level. Lower acridity levels decline your bet of future kidney stones.

Pomegranate juice's effect on preventing kidney stones ought to be better thought of, but considering a 2014 animal review, there could be some benefit in taking pomegranate eliminate. In the audit, it cut down the bet of stones.

It's not palatable how much pomegranate juice you can safely drink throughout the span of the day, yet a serving or two consistently is conceivable reasonable for a considerable number individuals.

The American Stroke Affiliation observes that a couple of drugs used to cut down cholesterol could interface with pomegranate juice. If you're taking any prescriptions, talk with an expert preceding endeavoring pomegranate juice.

### 2. Kidney bean stock

The stock from cooked kidney beans is a standard dish, often used in India. Certain people ensure that it can chip away at urinary and kidney prosperity, but there's little verification to say whether this fix is strong. To endeavor it, basically strain the liquid from cooked beans and drink it a couple of times every day.

**Other standard fixes**

The going with home fixes could contain trimmings that aren't at this point in your kitchen. You should have the choice to get them from your local prosperity food store or on the web.

### 3. Dandelion

The dandelion plant has for quite a while been used as a stomach related help. Various bits of the plant are made sure to help with clearing out waste, increase pee yield, and further foster ingestion. Dandelions have supplements A,

B, C, and D and minerals like potassium, iron, and zinc.

One lab study showed that dandelion is convincing in hindering the advancement of kidney stones. Anyway, these results are from lab tests, and there's little evidence to say whether dandelion works the same way when consumed by people. Human assessments are supposed to check whether it's a safeguarded and effective fix.

You can make new dandelion juice from the plant's leaves or buy the roots as a tea or concentrate.

Accepting you make it new, you may in like manner add orange strip, ginger, and apple to taste.

While restricted amounts of dandelion are likely safe for considerable number individuals, it's not understood whether consuming dandelion things in tremendous sums is secured. Certain people can be oversensitive to dandelion, especially expecting you have aversion to ragweed, marigolds, chrysanthemums, or daisies.

High doses of dandelion may be unsafe for people with explicit clinical issue, **for instance,**

- heart conditions
- high or low heartbeat
- liver or kidney conditions
- diabetes
- growing

Visit with an expert before taking dandelion root remove, as it can interface for specific medications. Accepting that you're taking diuretics, dandelion is routinely not proposed.

### 4. Wheatgrass juice

Wheatgrass is stacked with various enhancements and has for a long while been used to further develop prosperity. Wheatgrass increases pee stream to help with passing the stones. It also contains basic enhancements that help with cleansing the kidneys.

You can drink 2 to 8 ounces of wheatgrass squeeze every day. To thwart coincidental impacts, start with the most diminutive aggregate possible and step by step move continuously up to 8 ounces.

In case new wheatgrass juice isn't available, you can acknowledge powdered wheatgrass supplements as facilitated.

Taking wheatgrass while starving can reduce your bet of nausea. On occasion, it could cause hunger adversity and blockage.

## 5. Horsetail

Horsetail is used as a diuretic to increase pee stream. It has antibacterial and cell support properties that could uphold as rule prosperity. It could in like manner decrease aggravation. Completely, these effects could really help your body with flushing out kidney stones.

The European Affiliation's European Solutions Office observes that horsetail should not be used by people with serious heart or kidney conditions. It's doable to have stomach related coincidental impacts while using horsetail and awareness's have moreover been represented.

Horsetail isn't recommended for young people or people who are pregnant, breastfeeding, or chest taking care of.

### When to see a subject matter expert

See an expert if you can't pass your stone in that frame of mind than about a month and a half or you begin experiencing outrageous secondary effects that **include:**

- serious desolation
- blood in your pee

- fever
- chills
- disorder
- disgorging

An expert will choose if you maintain that medication or some other treatment should help you with passing the stone.

**The primary concern**

In spite of the way that it very well may be abnormal, it's doable to pass a kidney stone in isolation.

You can take command over-the-counter (OTC) pain relievers to diminish any disturbance you could understanding. These consolidate acetaminophen (Tylenol), ibuprofen (Advil), or naproxen (Aleve).

Make sure with continue to comply to an expert's rules until the stone passes, and don't drink alcohol.

At the point when you pass a kidney stone, you could have to save it to take to an expert for testing. To save the stone, you need to strain your pee.

You can do this by using a pee screen, which you can get from the expert's office. An expert can sort out what kind of stone it is and help with encouraging an assigned contravention plan.

Talk with an expert about lifestyle changes you can make to help with holding extra stones back from outlining. Consistently check in with an expert before endeavoring home fixes, flavors, or improvements.

Flavors aren't coordinated for quality and goodness by the Food and Prescription Association (FDA), so research your choices and focal points for acquirement.

Another examination of 27 extraordinary upgrades for kidney prosperity viewed that as 66% of them included trimmings that have no assessment to help their use.

# CHAPTER SEVEN

## STRATEGIES FOR PREVENTING KIDNEY STONES

We integrate things we accept are useful for our perusers. If you buy through joins on this page, we could secure a little commission Here's our cycle.

### Kidney stone expectation

Kidney stones are hard mineral stores that design inside your kidneys. They cause horrible desolation when they go through your urinary part.

Up to 12 percent of Americans are influenced by kidney stones.

Likewise, at whatever point you've had one kidney stone, you half will undoubtedly get another inside the accompanying 10 years.

There's no one certain strategy for preventing kidney stones, especially if you have a family foundation of the condition. A mix of diet and lifestyle changes, as well as specific medications, may help with reducing your bet.

### The best strategy to hinder kidney stones typically

Rolling out little improvements as per your continuous eating routine and food plan could go very far toward preventing kidney stones.

### 1. Stay hydrated

Drinking more water is the best method for thwarting kidney stones. In case you don't drink enough, your pee result will be low. Low pee yield infers your pee is more thought and less leaned to crumble pee salts that cause stones.

Lemonade and crushed orange are furthermore incredible decisions. Both of them contain citrate, which could hold stones back from outlining.

Endeavor to drink around eight glasses of fluids consistently or enough to pass two liters of pee. If you exercise or sweat an incredible arrangement, then again in case you have a past loaded up with cystine stones, you'll require additional fluids.

You can sort out whether or not you're hydrated by looking at the shade of your pee — it should be clear or light yellow. In case it's dull, you truly need to drink more.

## 2. Eat more calcium-rich food sources

The most notable sort of kidney stone is the calcium oxalate stone, convincing numerous people to figure they should do whatever it takes not to eat calcium. The converse is substantial. Low-calcium diets could assemble your kidney stone bet and your bet of osteoporosis.

Calcium supplements, in any case, may fabricate your bet of stones. Taking calcium supplements with a supper could help with decreasing that bet.

### 3. Eat less sodium

A high-salt eating routine extends your bet of calcium kidney stones. According to the Urology Care Foundation, a great deal of salt in the pee holds calcium back from being reabsorbed from the pee to the blood. This causes high pee calcium, which could incite kidney stones.

Eating less salt associates keep pee calcium levels lower. The lower the pee calcium, the lower the bet of making kidney stones.

To diminish your sodium utilization, read food names circumspectly.

**Food assortments renowned for being high in sodium include:**
- dealt with food assortments, similar to chips and wafers
- canned soups
- canned vegetables

- lunch meat
- sauces
- food assortments that contain monosodium glutamate
- food assortments that contain sodium nitrate
- food sources that contain sodium bicarbonate (baking pop)

To improve food sources without using salt, endeavor new flavors or a sans salt, local getting ready blend.

## 4. Eat less oxalate-rich food sources

Some kidney stones are made of oxalate; a trademark compound found in food sources those dilemmas with calcium in the pee to shape kidney stones. Limiting oxalate-rich food sources could help with holding the stones back from forming.

**Food sources high in oxalates are:**

- spinach
- chocolate
- sweet potatoes
- coffee
- beets

- peanuts
- rhubarb
- soy things
- wheat grain

Oxalate and calcium integrate in the gastrointestinal framework before showing up at the kidneys, so it's harder for stones to approach if you eat high-oxalate food assortments and calcium-rich food assortments all the while.

## 5. Eat less animal protein

Food assortments high in animal protein are acidic and may augment pee destructive. High pee destructive could cause both uric destructive and calcium oxalate kidney stones.

**You should endeavor to confine or avoid:**

- burger
- poultry
- fish
- pork

## 6. Avoid L-ascorbic corrosive upgrades

L-ascorbic corrosive (ascorbic destructive) supplementation could cause kidney stones, especially in men.

According to one 2013 review, men who took high doses of L-ascorbic corrosive upgrades duplicated their bet of molding a kidney stone. Investigators don't actually acknowledge that L-ascorbic corrosive from food conveys a comparative bet.

### 7. Explore local fixes

Chanca Piedra, generally called the "stone breaker," is a renowned normal individual's answer for kidney stones. The zest is made sure to help with hindering calcium-oxalate stones from molding. Reducing the size of existing stones is similarly acknowledged.

# CHAPTER EIGHT

## WAYS OF THWARTING KIDNEY STONES WITH MEDICATION

On occasion, switching up your dietary choices may not be adequate to hinder kidney stones from molding. Expecting you have dull stones, talk with your essential consideration doctor about which occupation medication can play in your balance plan.

### 1. Till your doctor about the medications you're at this point

Taking explicit arrangements or non-physician endorsed

medications can achieve kidney stones.

**A part of these medications are:**

- decongestants
- diuretics
- protease inhibitors
- anticonvulsants
- steroids
- chemotherapy drugs
- uricosuric meds

The more you consume these meds, the higher your bet of kidney stones. Accepting at least for now that you're taking any of these medications, banter with your PCP about other remedy decisions. You shouldn't stop ingesting any embraced medications without your essential consideration doctor's underwriting.

## 2. Letting your doctor about security medicines

Accepting at least for now that you're leaned to explicit sorts of kidney stones, certain prescriptions can help with controlling how much that material present in your pee. The kind of solution embraced will depend upon the sort of stones you typically get.

**For example:**

In case you get calcium stones, a thiamine diuretic or phosphate may be useful.

If you get uric destructive stones, allopurinol (Zyloprim) can help with decreasing uric destructive in your blood or pee.

Expecting you get struvite stones, long stretch enemy of contamination specialists may be used to help with diminishing how much organisms present in your pee

Kidney stones can cause a couple of gastrointestinal secondary effects, as well as GI disarrays that warrant a trip to an expert's office.

Kidney stones are hard, set masses that can approach in your kidneys.

They're typical, affecting around 600,000 Americans reliably. While anyone can have kidney stones, different sorts of stones are essentially inclined to impact different social occasions.

There are many reasons you could have kidney stones. A couple of sorts of stones are achieved by genetic conditions. Others are associated with stomach related issues, not taking in a satisfactory number of fluids, and certain illnesses.

Kidney stones are connected with outrageous torture in your waist, lower back, and sides anyway they can cause various issues moreover.

Kidney stones have an incredible connection with your gastrointestinal structure. We ought to examine what the two could mean for each other.

### Will kidney stones cause gastrointestinal incidental effects?

Right when you have a kidney stone, a part of the secondary effects that you first warning might be associated with your gastrointestinal structure.

### Torture

Gastrointestinal distress is the most well-known result of kidney stones. It's every so often called renal colic.

This kind of exacerbation every now and again goes this way and that in waves, and it regularly feels sharp and outrageous. You could feel it in your mid-district, sides, lower back, and groin.

### Nausea

Kidney stones can similarly incite squeamishness, a portion of the time as a reaction to torture. This incidental effect isn't exactly essentially as typical as torture it, and may show that you truly need speedy clinical thought.

## Heaving

Heaving can in like manner be a symptom of kidney stones, but like squeamishness; it's one of the more surprising incidental effects. If you acknowledge kidney stones are the justification behind your hurling, bring an expert right.

## Expected gastrointestinal intricacies of kidney stones

The gastrointestinal results of kidney stones depicted above are things that could make you mindful of a kidney stone. Incidental effects regularly vanish after the kidney stones are managed.

Due to having kidney stones, you could in like manner experience new gastrointestinal issues.

**Prickly entrail condition**

A concentrate in Taiwan saw that adults will undoubtedly cultivate testy stomach condition (IBS) following having a kidney stone. More than 30% of new occasions of IBS occurred in the range of a half year following having a stone strangely.

### Entrail obstacle

While it's exceptionally unprecedented, a 2013 case report portrayed a more settled female whose kidney stone caused a stomach obstruction. This provoked disarrays that are not generally associated with kidney stones, including absolute stopping up and feculent hurling.

### Might gastrointestinal issues anytime cause kidney stones?

Kidney stones can cause gastrointestinal incidental effects and complexities, yet is the opposite substantial as well? As it turns out, for sure, a couple of gastrointestinal issues can provoke kidney stones.

## Detachment of the entrails

The runs have many causes and are depicted by watery strong releases that are unending and sincere. A short episode of free entrails is likely not going to cause kidney stones. Steady free guts, regardless, can incite absence of hydration, which is one of the known explanations behind kidney stones.

# CHAPTER NINE

## PROVOCATIVE INSIDE CONTAMINATION

Provocative inside contamination (IBD) implies a social event of issues that impact your stomach related organs and gastrointestinal framework, including ulcerative colitis and Crohn's disorder. The disturbance related with these conditions can make it hard for your body to suitably ingest explicit blends. This malabsorption can every so often cause kidney stones to shape.

### Stomach operations

On occasion, stomach operations like gastric diversion and sleeve operations can cause issues like free entrails or malabsorption. As depicted over, these issues truly might conceivably incite kidney stones.

## Other kidney stones incidental effects

There are a couple of results of kidney stones that don't impact your gastrointestinal structure. Accepting you have kidney stones, you could experience some, all, or none of these aftereffects. Simply an expert can dissect kidney stones, so if you're unsure, you should consult with an expert about your incidental effects.

Kidney stone secondary effects that are not gastrointestinal **include:**

- anguishing pee
- persistent or basic pee
- appalling pee
- horrendous smelling pee
- obscure pee
- inconvenience peeing
- fever
- chills
- sweating

**When to contact an expert if you expect you have kidney stones**

The most un-prominent treatment for kidney stones is to permit them to pass ordinarily isolated by leaving your body with your pee. Nonetheless, occasionally, your kidney stones might be excessively enormous to safely pass isolated. Expecting that left untreated, this could cause a check. The most ideal way to know if a stone is adequately little to give its own is to have it reviewed by a trained professional.

The most notable result of kidney stones is torture, yet anguish can be achieved by various conditions. If you figure you could have a kidney stone, it is ideal to call a specialist.

If you experience other gastrointestinal issues, for instance, infection or hurling, it could mean your kidney stone is more limit. For this present circumstance, surely stick out.

**Frequently looked for explanation on certain things**

The association between kidney stones and gastrointestinal issues is amazing, with each having the option to create the other in unambiguous circumstances. Here are answers to the most generally perceived requests regarding this matter.

## Can kidney stones impact strong releases

While this is the kind of thing that could happen, overall the reaction is no. Kidney stones don't usually impact strong releases other than in exceptionally phenomenal cases, for instance, a kidney stone causing an entrail deterrent.

## What GI issues can cause kidney stones?

Parchedness and malabsorption can both lead to kidney stones. Both of these issues can be achieved by GI issues including:

- consistent free entrails

- provocative stomach infection
- stomach operations

## What GI issues can kidney stones cause?

Adults who have their most noteworthy kidney stone will undoubtedly cultivate disagreeable entrail issue inside the going with a half year than adults who have never had a kidney stone.

## Could kidney stones cause IBS?

While it's not known whether kidney stones can cause IBS, adults who have had a kidney stone will undoubtedly encourage

IBS throughout the accompanying a half year than individuals who haven't. More investigation is at this point expected to conclude whether kidney stones can directly cause IBS.

www.ingramcontent.com/pod-product-compliance
Lightning Source LLC
Chambersburg PA
CBHW071213240526
45470CB00018B/1819